The Metamorphosis:
21 Days to A New You

Dr. Sierra Bizzell

Dedication:

I want to first say thank you to The Most High God for allowing me to make it through yet another year and realize all of my wildest dreams.

To my husband and my coach: Thanks for pushing me to be better and strive for greater even when I don't think that I'm ready or prepared. I love you and you will forever be my hero and my inspiration.

To my parents: I love you so much! Thank you for always supporting me and being my biggest cheerleaders.

To my children: You're the most amazing people that I know and I love you three more than you will ever know.

Contents

Introduction

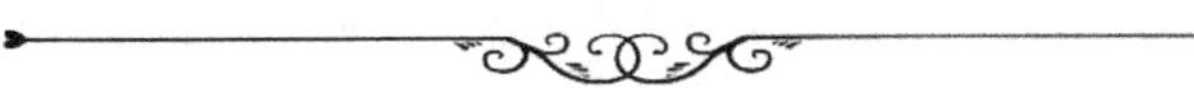

Hi! My name is Dr. Sierra Bizzell and I want to welcome you to my 21 day program. I hold a PhD. in Leadership, but more importantly I am here to help you become a new version of yourself. I am a Certified Doula, Health Coach, Master Herbalist and I'm currently studying to be a Doctor of Natural Medicine. I have been studying health, diet, herbs, and supplements for over 10 years and I am excited to share this program with you.

I started on this journey 10 years ago when my body went haywire after the birth of my oldest daughter. I spent hundreds of dollars buying programs, talking to health coaches, reaching out to natural doctors, seeing massage therapists, trying herbs, and did countless hours of research trying to heal.

One night while I was in my bed in excruciating pain, I cried out to God and told him that if he helped me to heal, then I would help others to do the same. Not too long after that, I figured out what needed to be done in order to heal myself from the issues that plagued me and today I am healthy and thriving!

I believe that it is my divine calling to dedicate my life to helping people heal so that they can truly live their best life right now. I'm so happy that you have decided to try my program and I can't wait to see what you will accomplish over the next 21 days!

Why metamorphosis? In my personal opinion, nature is beautiful. It holds the keys to the secrets of the universe that man has been trying to understand for many years. It is a constant reminder that there is something greater than all of us and it shows us that we are just a small part of something greater. Many people love to watch the butterfly as it soars around in the air seemingly without a care in the world, but no one tends to think of the process that it had to go through to get there.

Metamorphosis requires change. It begins with a state of youthful immaturity and ends in something great. I want to take you from where you are right now in a state of uncertainty and lack of direction, into the person that you have always dreamed of becoming. It is my hope that reading this one book will be the catalyst that will change your life!

This program was designed to change your life! So whether young or old, man or woman, you will find practical applications for your life that are attainable and easy to implement.

Now don't get my wrong, there will be days when you will want to quit, there will be times when you have to dig deep, but if you stick with it, the results will be worth every bit of discomfort that you may experience. I am here to help you and guide you along this journey, so feel free to reach out to me via email at sierra.beautifulbeginnings@gmail.com.

Let's get started!!!

Stage 1—-The Egg

Chapter 1: Goal Setting

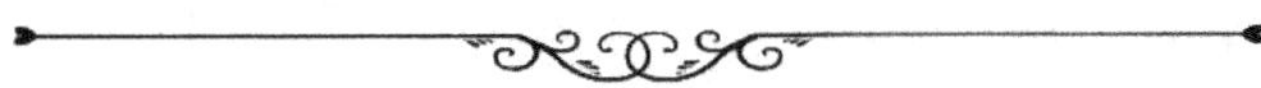

"By recording your dreams and goals on paper, you set in motion the process of becoming the person you most want to be. Put your future in good hands: your own."

~Mark Victor Hansen

Day 1:

Welcome to day 1 of the program. Today you are in the egg stage of your journey. You're at the very beginning of this process and filled with potential that you have yet to reach.

In this first phase I will hold your hand as if you're a newborn being given milk, but as you continue throughout this process, more of the responsibility will be placed upon you. For now let's focus on your very first task.

Most people have goals. However, most of those goals are either long-term goals that have no action plan tied to them, or they are short-term goals that do not benefit the future of the individual. In fact, when my clients come to see me, they just want results, but they think that you can somehow reach that desired result without a plan.

As a health coach, it is my job to assist my clients in not only reaching their end goal, but also to set a plan in place so that they have a step by step guide to navigate their path toward meeting that goal. Without a clear plan, most of our goals are destined to fail before they even begin. Therefore, it is important that we take the time to really work on defining our goals and creating a step by step plan to implement the goal.

Some people simply want to lose weight. However, when a goal isn't clearly defined, then you really just have a wish. Let me explain a little further. If my goal is to lose weight, but I have not set a specific "goal weight", then I'm probably not going to lose weight because I have nothing to aim for. However, if I say that my goal is to lose 10 pounds, then I have a clear goal and I'm more likely to work towards reaching that goal weight.

Step 1 on this 21 day journey is to come up with your goals. I want to get healthier isn't really a goal! I need to know what problem you want to solve so that we can create a clear action plan on how to get there.

Today I want you to take the time to clearly define your goals. Take the time to write down your goals. Except this time MAKE IT PLAIN! Stop writing vague goals and write down exactly what you would like to achieve and the timeframe in which you want to achieve it. A wise person once said, "If your goals (dreams) don't scare you, then they're not big enough." Therefore, you should write down your deepest desires and dreams, but this time write them down with clear vision. You should be able to see your dreams so vividly that if you closed your eyes and imagined them, they would seem as if they were already real. Have faith in yourself and know that the goals that you have are attainable, but it's up to you to do the work to reach those goals.

Now I want to ask you a few questions to help you decide on your personal goal(s).

What are 2 goals that you have for your health? What are 2 goals that you have for your life?

____

____

____

____

____

____

____

Do you believe that your goals are clearly defined? Why or why not?

____

____

____

____

____

____

How can you better define your goals?

____

____

____

____

____

____

____

What are 3 things that you would like to gain from this program?

____

____

____

____

____

____

____

"Write the vision, and make it plain on tablets, that he may run that readeth it"

Habakkuk 2:2 ASV

"Thinking is easy, acting is difficult, and to put one's thoughts into action is the most difficult thing in the world."

~ Johann Wolfgang von Goethe

Day 2:

Now that we have written down your goals, it's time to explore the reasons why you have not been able to achieve these goals. Oftentimes we set goals that are vague, but we also lack an action plan. Have you ever sat down and figured out a true plan to achieve your goals?

If your goal is to go back to school, have you looked at programs, figured out the cost, looked at scholarships, talked to an advisor, decided on a major, etc?

If you want to lose weight, have you decided how much weight you want to lose, purchased a gym membership, hired a personal trainer, decided on a meal plan, and started planning out your meals for your diet? If not, the question is why haven't you taken any steps towards reaching your goals?

Maybe you tried in the past and failed, but that should not stop you from making your dreams a reality. Today's question is simply this…

What would it take for you to be able to reach your goals? Is it money that's stopping you? Is it having the free time? Is it fear? What is holding you back from reaching your goals?

____

____

____

____

____

____

____

____

Write down 3 things that it would take for you to reach your goals and take the first step to make that happen.

____

____

____

____

____

____

____

____

What steps can you take today to begin working on your goals?

____

____

____

____

____

____

____

____

Chapter 2: Clear Your Mind

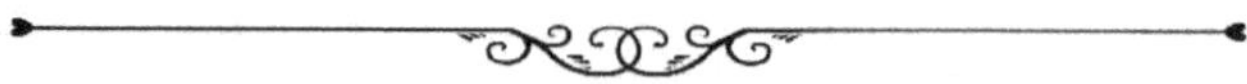

"You are who you are and what you are because of what has gone into your mind. You can change who you are and what you are by changing what goes into your mind"

~ Zig Ziglar

Day 3:

In 1992, En Vogue released a song called "Free Your Mind". The lyrics said, "Free your mind and the rest will follow..." This one line has so much wisdom in it because if your mind is clear, everything else will fall into place. The mind is so powerful that you can will yourself to be healed, cause yourself to fail, and even manifest sickness through your thoughts. Today's lesson is about clearing your mind so that you can heal it.

Healing your mind is essential to being successful in this challenge and in life. One way that we will do this is by learning to look at the negative thought patterns that we tend to have. Negative thoughts tend to become negative behaviors, so let's identify those thought patterns and learn to control them so that they don't control you!

If you are a person who says, "I don't have negative thoughts.", then you're totally lying to yourself. We all have them everyday and some of us have them more often than others. Today I want you to take a hard look at yourself.

What are those deep dark thoughts that you tend to try to push to the back of your mind? Maybe you tell yourself that you're not good enough. Maybe you tell yourself that you're a failure. Maybe you're afraid of success because someone told you that you would never be great. Whatever those negative thoughts are, I want you to bring them out to the surface, so that we can get rid of the blockages that they have been creating for you. Be real with yourself and dig up all of those thoughts that you tried to bury. It's time to remove the dead thoughts so that you can truly live!

Identifying your negative thoughts can really help you to shift your mindset. You must first know the problem in order to fix it. Just as a doctor must confirm a diagnosis before they start to treat an issue, it is important for you to identify your negative thoughts and the source of these thoughts before you can make changes.

Write down 3 negative thoughts that you had today.

____

____

____

____

____

____

What were you doing when you had those thoughts?

____

____

____

____

____

____

How did those thoughts affect you? What did they stop you from accomplishing?

____

____

____

____

____

____

"Attitude is a choice. Happiness is a choice. Optimism is a choice. Kindness is a choice. Giving is a choice. Respect is a choice. Whatever choice you make makes you. Choose wisely."

~ Roy T. Bennett

Day 4:

Now that you have identified your negative thought patterns, it is important that you learn to take those thoughts captive. Whenever you have a negative thought about yourself or your abilities, I want you to replace it with the following affirmation, "I can, I will, and I must succeed."

Doing this will help your subconscious mind to default to thinking positive thoughts instead of negativity. Overtime you will begin to notice a change in the way that you think and in the types of people that you attract.

When you live a life full of negativity, even the cells in your body become negative. Psychoneuroimmunology is a relatively new interdisciplinary field that studies how our thoughts and feelings influence our brain, nervous system, and disease-fighting mechanisms. In fact, it is believed that some of the health challenges that we have are not directly related to our genetic makeup or disposition, but rather they are a direct result of our thoughts and feelings (Brain, Behavior, and Immunity, 2007). Therefore, it is important that you watch your thoughts and feelings so that you can improve your overall health.

I want you to make it a habit to practice saying our new affirmation every time you have a negative thought about yourself. Keep practicing this until it becomes automatic! By replacing your negative self talk with positivity, you are rewiring your brain to default to a positive setting. While you won't always be positive, you will be in the habit of having positive beliefs about yourself and your ability to succeed. The more you speak it, the more you will become it! As we all know, "As a man thinketh, so is he!" (Proverbs 23:7)

How does saying this affirmation make you feel?

____

____

____

____

____

____

____

____

Do you believe that you can succeed? (Be sure to be really honest with yourself)

____

____

____

____

____

____

____

If not, where do you think these beliefs originated?

____

____

____

____

____

____

____

Chapter 3: Mind Body Connection

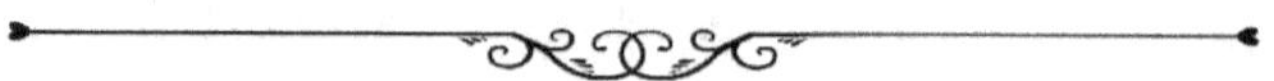

"Happier thoughts lead to essentially a happier biochemistry. A happier, healthier body. Negative thoughts and stress have been shown to seriously degrade the body and the functioning of the brain, because it's our thoughts and emotions that are continuously reassembling, reorganizing, re-creating our body."

~ Dr. John Hagelin

Day 5:

According to http://pne.people.si.umich.edu/kellogg/012.html, there is a correlation between watching television and one's overall mental health. What you watch has the ability to affect your intellectual development, increase your levels of anxiety, lead to depression, and induce aggressive behavior. Therefore, what you put into your mind may have a direct effect on your body and you should be careful about what you allow into your subconscious mind.

Not only does what we watch tend to affect our bodies, but what we listen to causes a similar reaction on the body as well.

When you listen to positive music, it evokes feelings of happiness and causes you to smile, but when you listen to sad and negative music, it has the opposite effect. According to Hans-Eckhardt Schaefer (2017), music can impact your body in ways that manifest physically. It can lead to anxiety, aggression, mental health challenges, etc.

Therefore, it is not only important to guard what you watch on television, but it's also important to make sure that you listen to things that are positive and uplifting most of the time. Just like everything else in life, balance is key and you don't want to put too much negativity into your subconscious mind because eventually, it will begin to manifest itself in your life.

Today I want you to take inventory of the things that you put into your subconscious mind. Think about the last 3 things that you've watched and listened to and answer the following questions.

Do you watch positive or negative shows? Why?

____
____
____
____
____
____
____

If you watch negative shows, do you think that it is affecting your overall well-being?

____

____

____

____

____

____

____

____

Today I want you to evaluate those who have the most influence on your life, are they positive or negative people? Why do you consider them to be positive or negative? If they are negative, then maybe it's time to re-evaluate those relationships or have a talk with them about their behaviors.

____

____

____

____

____

____

____

____

Day 6:

Heal your mind and your soul and you will have the body of your dreams.

~ Roxana Jones

Healing your body starts with the mind. Most people believe that diet and exercise is the most important part of the journey to health, but it's not. If your mindset isn't right, then you won't be able to eat well because you will fall back into your old habits. You must first decide to change your mindset and then change our health.

Think about it! How often have you started a diet or decided to change your lifestyle and then you did well for 3 weeks, but fell off the wagon?

Oftentimes when things get hard or they inconvenience us in any way, we quit! This is not because we are lazy, it's because our minds quit long before we tried to make a change. The difference in the people who succeed and those who fail is all in the mind.

Successful people are willing to do things that other people don't do because they have decided that their end goal is important enough not to quit. Those who succeed often listen to positive podcasts, read lots of inspirational books, hire coaches/mentors, and they listen to positive music. They rarely watch TV and when they do, they watch positive programs. Success begins in the mind, so today you're going to begin to cleanse your mind because this is the key to ensuring that you will be successful!

In order to cleanse the mind, you should be restricting the things that you allow into your innermost self.

For the next 3 days try not to listen to, watch, or read anything negative. Instead find positive shows to watch, uplifting music to listen to, and 1 inspirational book to read. This means avoiding shows that are filled with gossip such as Jerry Springer, the news which can be super depressing, some social media posts, and certain types of music.

Today make a list of 3 positive songs that you will listen to for the duration of this challenge.

____

____

____

____

____

____

____

After 3 days of taking in positivity, write about any changes that you have noticed within yourself. Discuss the changes that you have noticed within yourself.

____

____

____

____

____

____

____

____

Chapter 4: Diet and Exercise

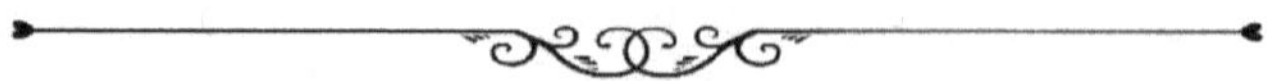

Larva Stage—

If you keep good food in your fridge, you will eat good food.

-Errick McAdams

Day 7:

Welcome to day 7! You've made it through 1 full week and it's now time to move on to a new stage of maturity. In the larva stage the insect is no longer a baby. They have moved through the early stages of life and this is the time in which they begin to ingest the food that they will need to complete their transformation.

You are now in this same stage of this program. You have learned everything that you need to know in order to prepare your mind for the next level, but now it's time to feed your body and your soul in preparation for the future.

Today we are going to talk about diet and exercise! What you eat is only a small portion of your diet, it's the emotions that are attached to eating that often cause problems. Most people are emotional eaters and they tend to eat when they feel sad or stressed.

We often see movies and tv shows where women are sitting in front of a big bowl of ice cream with tears rolling down her cheeks because she was dumped by her boyfriend. When people are sad or stressed they are more likely to pick up a box of cookies rather than eat a bowl of kale. That's why you need to understand emotions and how they relate to food.

If you can pinpoint why you eat the way you do, then you can begin to deal with the root cause of your food issues. I want you to pay close attention because people often assume that if you aren't overweight, you can't have food issues.

This couldn't be further from the truth! I would like to challenge this thought by saying that I believe most Americans have issues with food due to the way in which we are taught to eat.

Americans live to eat, but in other countries people are taught to eat to live. They cook fresh foods and they make dinner as a family. In America, people hate to cook. They enjoy eating fast meals, and they want to eat things that are filled with sugar and salt. Our diet causes death and food is supposed to help your body to thrive. It is important that you learn to control your eating habits and start managing your food emotions. Learn to eat based on what your body needs and not based on how you feel!

Today I want you to take a hard look at what you eat and why you eat it. This exercise will force you to really pay attention to your emotions. If at any point it becomes too emotional for you, take a deep breath and allow yourself to process what you're feeling and work through your emotions. The reason why you're choosing to eat certain foods when you're feeling emotional is because you never dealt with the root cause of the emotions, so it's time to really work through those issues.

Make a list of everything that you eat today. Note the time that you eat it and how you felt at that time.

____

____

____

____

____

____

____

____

Did you notice any patterns within your eating? If so, what are they?

____

____

____

____

____

____

____

Are you a stress eater or do you eat when you are sad or angry?

____

____

____

____

____

____

____

Think back to when you started this behavior. What kind of connection do you have with food? Is it a healthy connection? If not, why?

____

____

____

____

____

____

____

____

What are some other ways that you can deal with your feelings and emotions? Write down 2 alternatives so that you can use them to replace your emotional eating habits. Examples: Going to the gym, taking a long hot bath, or even going to therapy.

____
____
____
____
____
____
____

Day 8:

"The food you eat can be either the safest and most powerful form of medicine or the slowest form of poison."

~Ann Wigmore

This program is all about cleansing your entire body. Today I want you to really focus on your health. Oftentimes in our society we tend to focus on our career, our family, our friends, and creating wealth, but we must realize that our health is more important than all of those things. Without health we cannot enjoy the things that we love.

People thrive when they have a routine. Today I want to help you build a healthy daily routine. Since we have identified the negative thoughts and eating patterns that we have, it's time to break them and heal!

You have already received your diet plan and today I want you to go into your kitchen and get rid of all of the foods that aren't healing to your body. These things include:

1. Processed foods such as chips, candy, cookies, cakes, microwave popcorn, bacon, etc.
2. Sugary sodas and juices.
3. TV dinners, chicken nuggets, and fish sticks.
4. Apple Sauce
5. Canned Foods
6. Soy based foods
7. Canned meats and boxed meals

If it didn't come from a plant, tree, or directly from an animal, then it's probably not good for you! Try to focus on eating fresh fruits and vegetables and clean meats (hormone free) during this challenge. If you are plant based, avoid soy and other processed foods during the cleanse.

Morning Routine:

Begin your day by drinking 8-10 oz of warm water with lemon or lime

Take time to breathe and try to do 10 min or stretching during this time.

Groom Yourself

Eat a healthy breakfast or a smoothie

Lunch

Lunch should be your biggest meal of the day, but try not to eat things that will cause you to become tired and sluggish. You should eat some protein that is the size of the palm of your hand, 2-3 servings of vegetables, and a whole grain (preferably brown or wild rice).

Dinner:

Eat before 7pm (unless you have some sort of health condition that requires you to eat later)

Eat a smaller meal such as a salad and soup. Keep your evening meals small and simple so that you can sleep better & so that your body can detoxify itself while you are asleep.

Before you make the excuse that you cannot eat bigger lunches due to lack of time, try meal prepping on Sundays or bring lunches from home. Avoid the temptation to spend money on food by making sure that you have food on hand.

Snacks:

When you eat snacks you should be eating things such as fruit, smoothies, and nuts & seeds (unless you are allergic to them). Try to avoid eating prepackaged snacks (unless it's a bag of nuts or seeds with no added salt or oils) or some guacamole.

Do you have a food routine? What does it look like? Write down what you eat each day and what time you eat it.

____

____

____

____

____

____

____

How is the routine that I just gave you different and in what ways can it help you?

____
____
____
____
____
____
____

Day 9:

"Movement is a medicine for creating change in a person's physical, emotional, and mental states.

~Carol Welch

Exercise is something that most people either love or hate! Those who love it tend to exercise often and those who hate it, only do it when they have to. Exercise is great for the body because it allows you to control your weight, reduce your risk of heart disease, assist the body in managing blood sugar and insulin levels, remove toxins from the body, and much more.

Exercise is also a great way to reduce stress and it can help you to improve your mental health and mood. By exercising daily you slow down the aging process and increase your chances of living longer.

In order to help you exercise more often, I want to encourage you to take 15 min in the morning (or during your lunch break) and 15 min in the evening to exercise. Set a timer and do as many exercises as you can during that time or go for a walk.

Since mornings should be kept light and positive, begin your morning by stretching and breathing for 15 min. If you have the time, take a 15 min walk (especially during your lunch break).

In the evening, try to opt for low impact workouts. There are lots of free workouts on youtube and low cost workouts such as Brittne Babe's challenges or workouts made by Fitness Blender. These workouts will challenge you, but they will help you to get healthy and fit. When you want to quit, remember your why and keep going. Aim to move each day and keep a record of how long you work out each day.

Do you exercise? If not, what is stopping you from exercising?

____
____
____
____
____
____
____
____

What negative thoughts have you told yourself about exercise? List 3 negative thoughts that you have about exercise and 3 ways that you can change this attitude.

____

____

____

____

____

____

____

If you don't exercise at all, start with 10 min workouts each day. During your lunch break, try to walk up and down a flight of stairs or walk around the building. Gradually add 5 min each day until you work your way up to 30 min per day.

Chapter 5— Mindfulness

"The feeling that any task is a nuisance will soon disappear if it is done in mindfulness."

– *Thích Nhất Hạnh*

Day 10

Every system within our bodies is interconnected. Eating healthy and changing your mindset are just a small part on the grander scale of the healing process. Next, we must begin to address the issues that are plaguing the body by becoming more mindful of our inner self and our needs.

Mindfulness is defined as the state of being conscious or aware of something. In this case, mindfulness is being aware of your thoughts, feelings, your stressors, and learning to meet your own needs.

We often work very hard to meet the needs of others without taking the time to meet our own needs. Most of us are pouring from empty cups which leaves us with nothing else to pour into those around us.

Mindfulness is taking the time to be aware of YOU. Pay attention to your body because it will let you know what it needs. Oftentimes our bodies get ignored and we end up paying the consequences which can be anything from digestive issues to something more severe like a heart attack.

In fact, over 80% of Americans are thought to be suffering from adrenal fatigue and they have no clue that this is the cause of their underlying issues (Washington Post, 2013).. Adrenal fatigue happens when stress causes your adrenal glands to become exhausted and fatigued. Consequently, they become unable to produce adequate amounts of hormones that help regulate certain systems within the body.

Adrenal fatigue can lead to low energy levels, brain fog, salt cravings, anxiety, and much more. One way to combat adrenal fatigue is by doing things that will help your body to rest and become more in tune with itself. Learning to listen to your body can be the key to unlocking your overall health and repairing the damage that has been done to your body.

Today I want you to identify your ideas about yourself and what you deserve.

Do you think mindfulness is important? Why or why not?

____

____

____

____

____

____

____

In what ways do you focus on yourself each week? When was the last

time that you did something for you?

____

____

____

____

____

____

____

Day 11

"Mindfulness is a way of befriending ourselves and our experience."

— *Jon Kabat-Zinn*

Mindfulness is more than just lighting some candles and going to bed at 9pm. It's more about the way that you treat yourself and how you let others treat you as well. It is knowing how to say no to things that don't serve you and not feeling bad or stressed for taking the time to take care of you.

Mindfulness requires us to have to become more aware of ourselves and the things that happen around us. In order to do this, we have to slow down and evaluate the connections that we have with those around us and ourselves. This can be hard because we don't like to sit still and "just be", but it is imperative for the health of our overall beings.

Here are 5 ways that you can reduce stress and become more mindful:

1. **Learn to accept yourself!** We as people tend to be overly critical of ourselves. Instead of focusing on the negatives, it is up to us to focus on positive things. Learn to celebrate your wins rather than always focusing on the things that you didn't do so well. This will help to improve our thoughts and in turn cause our bodies to become happier! Take 5 min each day and write down 5 wins that you had throughout the day.

2. **Take mini-breaks.** Most of us tend to take frequent breaks when working, but oftentimes we replace work with more work. We check our emails, respond to messages, and answer

phone calls. While all of this is fine, it can sometimes add to our stress levels rather than reducing it.

Instead of doing these things, try really taking a break. Take 2-3 min to relax without checking social media or looking at your phone. Instead use this time to allow yourself to refocus and get in tune with your body.

If your body is tired of sitting, stand up and stretch, take a few deep breaths, and then get back to work. Practicing mini-breaks can help you become more productive because you will spend more time working hard so that you can get to your next break! Aim to do this 2-3 times per day if you can.

3. **Live in the moment.** As people we live in the future. We're always thinking about what's next, what we need to get done, writing a to-do list for the next day, and trying to plan for the weeks and months ahead. However, sometimes it's necessary to stop and think about the present.

   When we learn to live in the present and truly be grateful for what we have now, then we will learn to truly find value in our lives. Try taking one evening each week and practice putting down the phone, turning off the television, and sitting down to dinner with your friends or family. Listen to what they have to say and really engage with them. Learn to value the present because the future isn't promised!

4. **Take a walk!** Walking is good for your health and it is extremely therapeutic. Walking without distractions allows us to become in tune with our thoughts and really be able to pay attention to our hearts desires. During this time you may get some of your most amazing ideas or be able to find the solutions to problems that you couldn't find before due to all of the things that tend to cloud our minds throughout the day. Take a 30 min walk each day (or at least 3 times per week) without distractions and really listen to your inner thoughts.

5. **Focus on your breath.** Deep breathing does amazing things for your body! Most of us have very shallow breaths and we don't ever take the time the focus on how we breathe because it happens automatically. Deep breathing allows you to relax, reduce cortisol levels, and lower your heart rate. Some studies have shown that this type of breathing can help you to reduce blood pressure as well. Take 2-3 min each day to focus on your breath. Doing this before bed can help you sleep better and relax your mind so that you fall asleep faster.

This can be done while sitting or laying down in your bed. Take a deep breath and hold it for 7 seconds and let it out slowly (count to 7 while letting it out). Repeat for 2-3 min each night and reap the benefits!!!

Which of these exercises would you like to try? How do you think it will benefit you?

____

____

____

____

____

____

____

____

Chapter 6— Connecting to your higher power

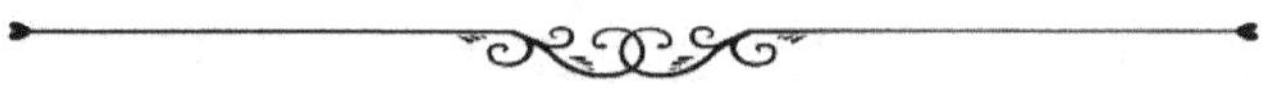

"There is no greater gift than realizing the constant presence of the Divine and His Absolute Power to create and restore all things."

— *Marta Mrotek*

The Pupa Stage——-

Day 12

Welcome to day 12! This is the beginning of the 3rd stage of this program. In the pupa stage the insect stops eating and begins to prepare for transformation. It during this time in which the caterpillar begins to focus on inward change.

In this stage of the program, I really want you to focus on you. It's time to dig deep and really look within for the answers that you seek. This part of the program will be difficult and if you stick with it, it will produce results.

This book is not in any way religious, but I do want to talk about the importance of a connection with a higher being. It is not my job to tell you what to believe, but rather to tell you that this connection is important because it is the only way that you can connect to your higher self. My higher power happens to be the God of the bible. While your higher power may be something different, you need to understand that every human has a divine understanding that there is some force that is greater than themselves and they seek to connect to this source.

By connecting to a higher power, we learn more about ourselves and our capabilities, and we are able to really gain insight into what we were created to be and do. One way that we can connect to a higher power is to use the art of meditation.

What is meditation?

Meditation is a practice that has been used by many different cultures for many different years. The term "meditation" stems from the latin term *meditatum,* which means "to ponder". Meditation happens when we allow ourselves to be at peace and we begin to ponder over our thoughts. It is my personal belief that trying to cause your mind to become blank doesn't really allow people to truly relax. In fact, the more you try to quiet your mind, the more you start to focus on quieting your mind than trying to focus on your thoughts. Instead, it is more important to focus on our thoughts and explore why we may be thinking certain things.

When you allow yourself to enter a space of being relaxed and in tune with your thoughts, you begin to allow yourself to hear from your higher being. Oftentimes the ideas and thoughts that you have during this time will seem as if they are divinely inspired and may be exactly what you need to help you get to the next level in life.

Many people don't meditate because they believe that it requires them to sit in a candlelit room in a criss cross applesauce posture, but this couldn't be further from the truth. Meditation can happen anywhere and at anytime. All you have to do is allow yourself to become intune with what you're thinking.

Today I want to encourage you to take the time to meditate and listen to what THE higher power is trying to say. Is there a solution that you need to find, an idea that you're trying to develop, or some emotion that you need to work through. If so, I encourage you to take 10 min to tune into your thoughts and begin to think about a problem that you need to solve. If you allow yourself to focus on that thought, then the solution will come.

Mental blocks to meditation

Some of us have been taught that meditation is spooky or weird. There are many different types of meditation and most religious texts discuss it in some form or fashion. Try to find out what you believe about meditation and how that relates to the way that you meditate. If you have been taught that one form of meditation is evil, then focus on the type of meditation that you find acceptable.

What are your thoughts on meditation? What are some mental blocks that could be keeping you from meditating?

____

____

____

____

____

____

____

Do you have a deep connection with your higher power? How is your connection (or lack thereof) affecting your life?

____

____

____

____

____

____

____

Day 13

"Faith in a higher power helps us to control our mind and thoughts."

–Mata Amritanandamayi

What is a higher power?

This question is totally personal, but it is my belief that a higher power is something higher than yourself. It is in everything and nothing can exist apart from it. When we realize that the greatest force in the universe, the one that created the entire galaxy, and the energy that causes everything to function is in us as well, then and only then do we begin to understand who we are.

The key to tapping into this higher power isn't crying on an alter, but really taking the time to connect with this great force. By understanding how great this force is and reverencing this higher being as something so powerful that it cannot be contained, you will really begin to look at the world around you differently.

When you begin to understand the creative power that is possessed within nature flows through your veins, then you begin to understand the power that is within you! You are filled with the same power that created the stars! If this power can create the stars, then it can certainly help you to create a better and more productive life.

Take time to really sit and think about how vast this universe is. Think about how wide the ocean is and how it can't be contained. Think about how powerful storms are and how they cannot be controlled. Now, I want you to think about yourself and how well designed your body is. If your body houses the force of such a powerful entity, then why aren't you treating it like that? Why aren't you feeding your body the things that it needs in order to function at its highest potential? Why aren't you feeding your mind the things that it needs to create amazing ideas by reading books and spending time in meditation? Why aren't you living up to the potential that you have?

Today I want you to tap into this power. You can call it prayer. You can call it setting intentions. You can call it talking to your higher self. Whatever it is that you believe, I want you to take the time to truly allow yourself to feel the presence of this great being. Talk to this higher power and allow it to speak to you. Even if you haven't been to a religious institution in years, take the time to really connect. Sit down and pour out your heart. Allow yourself to talk openly about your struggles. If you don't feel comfortable talking, then write them down.

Next take the time to really think about the greatness that lives inside of you and what you can accomplish. Do not allow self doubt to enter your mind. Instead, repeat your affirmation that we talked about earlier in this book and allow yourself to be open to the possibilities.

What did you learn about yourself during this exercise?

____

____

____

____

____

____

____

____

How did it feel to truly connect to your higher power? What was stopping you from connecting before?

____

____

____

____

____

____

____

____

Chapter 7: Resting and Unplugging

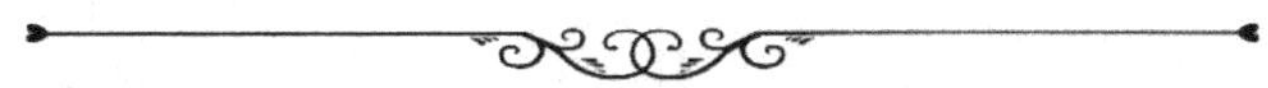

Day 14 Resting

"Sleep is the best meditation."

– Dalai Lama

According to most physicians rest is an essential part of healing the body (CDC, 2019). Getting an adequate amount of sleep allows the body's blood pressure to regulate itself, helps lower the chances of weight gain, improves concentration and productivity, decreases one's risk of heart disease, and minimizes your chances of developing type 2 diabetes.

Research has shown that those who do not get adequate amounts of sleep often have higher risks of depression and impared immune functioning. Therefore, it is extremely important to get enough rest each night. Since some people work weird hours and do not have consistent sleep schedules, it is important that they allow their bodies to rest 1 day per week.

Many ancient cultures such as the Jews and Babylonians implemented a practice in which they rested for 24 hours each week. During this time they did not do ANY work such as housework, working at their jobs, or traveling for long distances. This is a practice that has continued to be practiced by Jews and it is said to be very good for the body. While I understand that it may not be possible to take a full 24 hour rest period each week, it is important to be sure that you take the time to relax each week and allow your body to rest.

Choose one day per week and try to RELAX. Lay down, watch tv, and sleep as much as you can. Doing this will help to improve you to rest and allow your body to heal. If you work a second or third shift job, be sure to purchase blackout curtains so that you can get more restful sleep. Sleeping in a room without light helps your body to get more restful sleep by tricking your brain into thinking that it's dark outside and allowing you to sleep for longer periods of time.

*Note: If you are like me and you have young children, try to do things with them that will cause them to rest. Watch movies together, take a family nap, walk together, and just enjoy the company of your children.

In order to get more sleep try the following:

1) Go to bed before 10:30pm (If you work 1st shift)

2) Aim to get at least 7 hours of sleep each night

3) Turn off all devices at least 1 hour before bed

4) Choose 1 day each week and rest as much as you can

How long do you sleep each night? How many times per week do you sleep for at least 7 hours?

____

____

____

____

____

____

____

How do you think this lack of sleep is affecting your body? Do you feel tired throughout the week? Do you often feel irritable?

____

____

____

____

____

____

____

Day 15 Unplugging

Especially when you have a lot going on, you must find a way to unplug and focus on yourself.

~Mandy Ingber

We live in a society that thrives on access to information. We have google, tv, radio, social media, and Youtube. Everywhere we go there are people giving us information and sometimes it can be overwhelming.

Statistics show that rates of depression, anxiety, and suicide are at an all-time high, but not many people understand what is happening. It is my belief that the cause of these issues is the time that we spend plugged into the matrix of life. We surf social media and watch television, rather than making genuine connections with our friends and family. We spend so much time seeing negative things, comparing ourselves to others, watching shows that make us feel inadequate, and we lack balance. These practices are horrible for our mental and physical well-being because there is no break from the constant emotional rollercoaster of life, but there is a solution.

One way to remedy this is to unplug ourselves for a few hours a week. This means staying off your phone, not watching television, and taking the time to fill your mind with positivity.

Many people will think that this idea is old school and that it is unnecessary, but this one simple act can help so much. The less time you spend filling your mind with negativity, the better you will feel.

Try unplugging each night beginning at 9:00pm. Instead of scrolling through social media before you go to sleep, spend time writing down the things that went well throughout the day, write about 3 things that you are thankful for, read something positive for 15 min, and meditate/practice deep breathing for 10 min. This one change in behavior can help to change your reality and allow your body to heal. Not only will you begin to feel better, but you will also notice that you will sleep better as well.

How many hours do you spend on social media each week?

____
____
____
____
____
____
____
____

Do you scroll through social media before you go to sleep? Do you think this affects the quality of your sleep?

____

____

____

____

____

____

____

____

Chapter 8: Self-Love and Self-Reflection

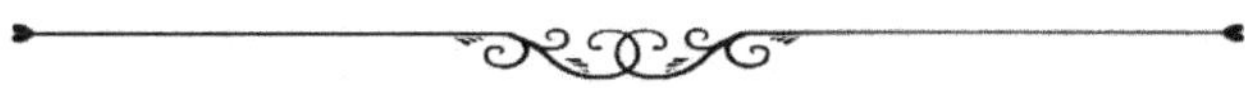

"Love yourself unconditionally, just as you love those closest to you despite their faults."

-Les Brown

Day 16: Self-love

We often hear songs on the radio such as Meghan Trainer's, "I Love Me", but how many of us actually love ourselves? Most of us believe that we love ourselves, but our actions do not reflect the love that we believe we have for ourselves. In fact, our actions often show that the opposite is true. We spend time eating foods that make our bodies feel sick, we have relationships with people that are toxic to our well-being, we do not exercise, we allow stress to overtake us, and we operate in a place of survival rather than thriving.

If you love another person, you do everything that you can in order to make that person feel as if they are loved. You check on that person, take care of them and try to help them maintain their health, you spend time with them, you make sure that they feel the love that you have for them through your actions. Yet, we do not do this for ourselves!

We have 1 body and our inner being is living within this body, but we are not loving our bodies, we are not treating ourselves with care, and we are creating an atmosphere of self-hate rather than self-love. You show how you feel about yourself through your actions. Therefore, the question becomes...do you really love yourself or are you tolerating yourself?

Self-love is defined as caring for one's own well-being and happiness while still caring about the well-being of others. Self-love does not mean that you are to become a narcissist. Rather, you learn to know your worth and you treat yourself accordingly.

Here are 5 ways to learn to love yourself:

1. Become mindful of your needs by learning to tune into your body. If you feel tired, allow yourself to rest rather than trying to push yourself to a point of exhaustion. Get to know yourself and ACT accordingly.

2. Practice self-care by doing things that help you to manage stress and feel happy. Take a long bath to relax, watch your favorite movie, get a massage, go for a walk, etc.

3. Set boundaries with others rather than saying yes to everything. It's ok to say no and you DO NOT have to feel bad about it.

4. Forgive yourself for all of your failures and work through the issues that you have. Seek therapy if it is necessary and work towards living in a place of being whole.

5. Live intentionally by setting goals and actually going for them. Stop sitting around waiting on happiness and do something that will allow you to live the life that you desire.

Do your actions reflect self-love?

____

____

____

____

____

____

____

____

In what ways can you improve the way that you treat yourself?

____

____

____

____

____

____

____

Day 17: Self- Reflection

"People who have had little self-reflection live life in a huge reality blind-spot."

— Bryant McGill

As people we tend to be unintentional hypocrites. We get upset about the actions of others, but we never take the time to look at ourselves. Instead we place the blame for all of our failures and mishaps on other people, but we never take responsibility for our own actions. While it is ok to acknowledge the part that others had to play in the things that went wrong in our lives, it is just as important to look at the places where we made mistakes so that we can improve our lives.

Self-reflection is not easy because it requires us to acknowledge our mistakes. It hurts because no one wants to admit their wrong doing, but it's necessary because it allows us to move from a place of being a victim and it helps us to avoid repeating the same mistakes. Self-reflection requires patience, growth, and maturity, and it is not for the faint at heart.

Here are 4 steps for self-reflection:

1. Take the time to think about a situation or experience. Write down what happened and how it made you feel.

2. Think about what you did during this situation or experience. What part did you play in the situation? Write down what you did and try not to focus on the things that others may have done.

3. Describe what you learned about yourself. Are you a person who gets angry quickly? Did you misunderstand what was said rather than taking the time to talk to the person?

4. Think about how you could have handled things differently. Write down ways that you would handle this situation if it were to happen again.

What did you learn about yourself during this exercise?

____

____

____

____

____

____

What things should you work on in order to ensure that this does not happen again?

____

____

____

____

____

____

____

Chapter 9: The Metamorphosis

"Metamorphosis is the most profound of all acts."

— *Catherynne M. Valente*

Metamorphosis

Day 18: Time for change

When we think of the word metamorphosis, we often think about butterflies this is the phase in which a butter matures from an egg to a full-grown adult butterfly and it is filled with many different stages. Just like a butterfly, you have been on the journey of change since the day you were born and it all leads to the day that you leave your former self behind and become the person that you were created to be.

Throughout this book you have been given strategies that will take you through a growth process. You began this book with a different mindset, a less than ideal diet, not a lot of direction, and you may not have been ready for the next level of life. Just like the larve, you were immature and you had a lot of growing to do, but now it's time to begin the process of change.

When a caterpillar is about to go through the process of becoming a butterfly, it often begins to do things differently. It eats differently, begins to seclude itself in its chrysalis and it starts to go through a transformation. When it is done, it emerges as something way more beautiful than anyone has ever seen.

This is your time of transformation within your chrysalis. It is time for you to take the necessary steps in order to create the metamorphosis that you desire to see. If you want change, you must first become the change that you desire. Therefore, it is time to take some steps in order to reach your goals.

Here are 3 signs that you're ready for change:

1. You are not happy with your current situation.
2. You notice that you are outgrowing some of the things that used to make you happy.
3. You have a desire to be great, but you don't know what to do.

If one or all of these signs apply to you, then it's time to make a change. In the next chapter, we will discuss ways to create a plan of action to lead you through this transitional phase and help you to emerge as a beautiful butterfly.

In what ways are you ready to change?

____

____

____

____

____

____

____

List 3 changes that you have made while reading this book?

____

____

____

____

____

____

____

Chapter 10- Creating a Plan

Plan your work and work your plan.

~Napoleon Hill

Day 19: Making Plans

Oftentimes we make plans and nothing happens. We write things down, create vision boards, read self-help books, and start exercise programs, but we never stick with them. Writing a vision is great. Visualizing the vision is awesome. Making plans is amazing, but it's the follow through that matters most.

In this chapter, I want to teach you how to create a fool-proof plan that will help you to finally become the change that you desire to see. In order to do this, you need to commit to this process for at least 21 days and understand that it takes at least 3 months to observe real change. When you begin to understand the process, then and only then will you stop quitting just because things got hard.

For most people change is cute. It's something that you say you want, but you never do what it takes to make it happen because it doesn't hurt enough. When you're sick enough, you will eat well and do what's necessary to become well. When you're broke enough, you will work hard and do whatever it takes to change your situation. The same thing goes for changing your lifestyle. Most people wait until they are at rock bottom before they change their actions.

Instead of hitting a rock bottom point, I want you to understand this one simple thing. Your life is either going to turn out well or turn out mediocre. It's up to you to decide.

The wealthy are wealthy for a reason. The fit are fit for a reason. The intellectuals are smart for a reason. It takes commitment to make changes and you need to commit to yourself. The same way that you don't quit on your job because it sucks is the same way that you need to treat yourself. If you can go to work every day knowing that your boss isn't great, your students will get on your nerves, and you won't get paid anything extra, you can do something that is going to change your life and actually make you better.

Here is my 7 step plan to get you to the life that you want now:

1. Make the decision to change and do it.---This is a lot harder than it seems, but the rewards are endless.

2. Decide on 1 thing that you want to improve.---Trying to do too many things will cause you to quit very quickly.

3. Do your research.--- It is important that you understand what it takes to reach your desired goal. Having the end goal and a time frame in mind will help you to prepare for the road ahead.

4. Hire a mentor--- Find someone who is doing the thing that you want to do and has been SUCCESSFUL in doing it. This may mean that you will have to pay them money to get their help, but investing in yourself is something that is necessary to reach the next level.

5. Stick to it for at least 3 months--- Establishing a new habit takes 21 days, but doing something for 3 months will help you to make it a part of your lifestyle.

6. Celebrate your wins--- Stop focusing on the things that you have not done well and celebrate all of your wins. This will help you to learn to focus on success rather than failure and create a mindset of success.

7. Keep going and DO NOT allow yourself to quit. It is easy to quit, but it's hard to keep going. No matter how hard things get, do not allow yourself to give up.

This may seem super simple. It may even sound easy or stupid, but it works. People all over the world are changing their lives and the lives of others by following this exact plan and it is working for them. The only thing standing in your way is you!

How many times have you started something and quit? How many goals has this stopped you from reaching?

____

____

____

____

____

____

____

What will you do differently this time to ensure that you succeed?

____

____

____

____

____

____

____

Chapter 11: Learning to be Grateful

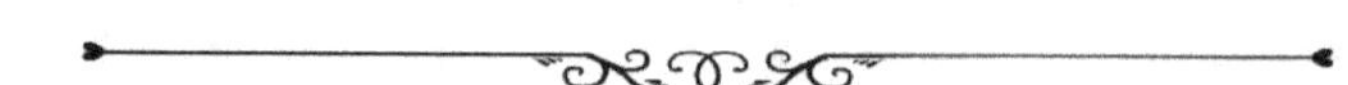

"Gratitude is a powerful catalyst for happiness. It's the spark that lights a fire of joy in your soul."

– *Amy Collette*

Day 20: Gratitude is THE Attitude

Gratefulness is something that most major religions and belief systems speak about. It is an attitude that many people do not have and without gratitude, we become unsatisfied with our current situation by always seeking something better. The problem with this is that when you are not thankful for what you have, you start to seek more and become envious of others.

In contrast, when you start to be grateful for even the small things, you will begin to see that abundance begins to flow to you. It's like having a bratty and spoiled child who is never happy with what they have and a child who is grateful for everything including the little things. Which child would you want to bless? If you want to attain wealth, better health, deeper relationships, you have to learn to give thanks for the things that you already have.

According to researchers (Allen, 2018), those who write down the things that they are thankful for each day are more satisfied with their lives, have an overall well-being, and a more positive mood. Other researchers found that those who practice gratitude even had less visitations to their physician (Harvard Medical School,n.d.). While one cannot say that there is a direct correlation between gratitude and health or happiness, the research indicates that it may have some effect on a person's well-being. Therefore, it is important to give thanks in everything!

What does it mean to be show gratitude? It means that you acknowledge that you have something and you allow yourself to truly feel as though you are happy about the things that you have been given. One way to do this is to take time each day to write down 7 things that you are thankful for. There are even notebooks, journals, and planners that allow you to show gratitude.

For the next 7 days, I want you to write down 7 things that you are grateful for each day. Allow yourself to truly feel thankful for these things no matter how bad your day may have been or what happened throughout the day. Find 7 things that you can write about each day, even if you have to be thankful for the basics such as food, water, clothes, air, life, health, and shelter. At the end of the 7 day period write about your thoughts in this exercise.

Do you feel that this exercise impacted your life?

____

____

____

____

____

____

____

What differences did you notice when you began to write about things that you are thankful for?

____

____

____

____

____

____

____

Chapter 12: Inspiration

"When I'm inspired, I get excited because I can't wait to see what I'll come up with next."

~Dolly Parton

Congratulations!! You made it to the very last day of this program. You have changed your mindset, worked on your eating habits, learned to take better care of yourself, and done the work to heal emotionally. Now it's time to get ready to transform.

Day 21: Be Inspired and Spread Your Wings

Today is the last day of this program! We have walked you through everything you need to know in order to change your life. We have taught you how to eat well, think better, treat yourself with kindness, take care of your body, connect to a higher power, and learn to love yourself. You have created goals, made a plan, and began working with a mentor who can help you to soar. Now it's time to emerge from your chrysalis, spread your wings, and fly!

This process is NOT easy, but the end goal is worth the struggle of change.

In order to stay on this path you need to be inspired. You will hit low points in life that will cause you to want to quit. People will say things to you that will break your spirit. You will want to throw in the towel because things overwhelm you, so you need to see others that are doing what you're doing. We would like to encourage you to join our fb group so that you can have accountability partners and people who understand what you're going through.

Without inspiration and people who are living the life that you want to live, you won't continue. When a person is training for a particular goal such as losing weight, gaining more muscle, etc., they often put up a picture of a person that they want to look like. I want to encourage you to find someone who is doing what you are doing and follow them on social media. Allow their path to inspire you to stay on your own path and aim to get to where you would like to be.

Do whatever it is that you need to do on this road so that you can get to your goals. Whatever you do...KEEP GOING, believe in yourself, and have faith in the abilities that were placed inside of you.

It's time to fly now and I hope that you continue on the path towards wholeness.

Name 3 people that inspire you.

____

____

____

____

____

____

____

Do you follow them on social media? If not, why aren't you following

them?

____

____

____

____

____

____

____

Are you ready to soar? If so, how does that make you feel?

____

____

____

____

____

____

____

What does soaring look like to you?

____

____

____

____

____

____

____

Thank you so much for joining me on this journey! I know that it hasn't been easy and that we have talked about a lot of issues that may have caused you to dig deep into the catacombs of your mind and open some old wounds. It is my hope that this book allows you to start your journey to creating the life that you want to live!

Be sure to follow me on social media:

- ➤ Facebook---- Sierrathebbdoula
- ➤ Instagram--- www.instagram.com/sierrathebbdoula
- ➤ Youtube: Sierrathebbdoula

May this book bring you health, wealth, and inspiration.

~Sierra

References:

https://www.health.harvard.edu/healthbeat/giving-thanks-can-make-you-happier

https://ggsc.berkeley.edu/images/uploads/GGSC-JTF_White_Paper-Gratitude-FINAL.pdf

https://exploreim.ucla.edu/mind-body/power-of-positivity/#science

https://www.washingtonpost.com/lifestyle/wellness/eat-right-sleep-tight-and-keep-life-from-pushing-your-buttons/2013/10/01/6907cc88-0c35-11e3-9941-6711ed662e71_story.html